Clear Acne Naturally

The Complete Guide to Acne-Free Skin with Proven Holistic Remedies, DIY Skincare Solutions, and Prevention Tips

Charles James

BONUS: Tips for sustaining clear skin after acne treatment.

Table of Contents

Chapter 1: Understanding Acne and Its Causes
1.1 Types of acne (blackheads, whiteheads, cystic acne).
1.2 Main causes of acne (hormones, diet, lifestyle, environment).
1.3 Why natural treatments work better for the skin.

Chapter 2: Natural Skincare Routines for Clear Skin
2.1 Daily and weekly skincare routines.
2.2 Skincare tips for different skin types (oily, dry, combination, sensitive).
2.3 Essential natural ingredients for clear skin.

Chapter 3: DIY Acne-Fighting Remedies
3.1 Face masks for acne-prone skin.
3.2 Simple recipes for natural toners and spot treatments.

3.3 How to exfoliate acne-prone skin gently.

Chapter 4: Healing Acne Scars Naturally
4.1 Types of acne scars (hyperpigmentation, pitted scars).
4.2 Natural remedies to fade scars (essential oils, gentle exfoliation).
4.3 Long-term healing and prevention of scars.

Chapter 5: Diet and Acne: Eating for Clear Skin
5.1 The gut-skin connection: How your diet affects your skin.
5.2 Foods to avoid that trigger acne.
5.3 Acne-fighting superfoods and their benefits.

Chapter 6: Daily Habits for Preventing Acne
6.1 The importance of hydration and its effect on skin.
6.2 How stress affects acne and natural stress-reduction techniques.
6.3 How sleep quality impacts skin health.

Chapter 7: Long-Term Skincare Maintenance

7.1 How to track your skin's progress and adjust your regimen.
7.2 Tips for sustaining clear skin after acne treatment.

Chapter 8: Natural Acne Treatments for Teens
8.1 Why teenage acne is different (hormones and puberty).
8.2 Simple, budget-friendly natural skincare for teens.
8.3 Teen diet tips for balancing hormones and reducing breakouts.

Chapter 1

Understanding Acne and Its Causes

1.1 Types of acne (blackheads, whiteheads, cystic acne)

Acne is a common skin condition that occurs when hair follicles become clogged with oil, dead skin cells, and bacteria. It usually affects areas like the face, back, chest, and shoulders. Acne can appear in various forms, each with different characteristics. Understanding the types of acne is essential to finding the right treatment and managing outbreaks effectively.

1. Blackheads

Blackheads are small, dark spots that appear on the skin's surface. They form when hair follicles become clogged with oil and dead skin cells but remain open. The dark color is not due to dirt but the result of the contents being exposed to air and oxidizing. Blackheads are non-inflammatory, meaning they don't cause swelling or pain, but they can still be persistent.

2. Whiteheads

Whiteheads are similar to blackheads, but in this case, the clogged pores remain closed. This creates small, white or flesh-colored bumps on the surface of the skin. Like blackheads, whiteheads are non-inflammatory but can become irritated if picked or squeezed. Whiteheads are often caused by the same factors that lead to blackheads—excess oil and dead skin cells trapped in the pores.

3. Cystic Acne

Cystic acne is a severe form of acne that occurs when pores become deeply clogged and inflamed. Unlike blackheads and whiteheads, cystic acne causes large, painful, pus-filled lumps beneath the surface of the skin. It often results in redness and swelling and can lead to scarring if not treated properly. Cystic acne is usually caused by hormonal imbalances and requires more aggressive treatment, such as prescription medications.

Understanding these different types of acne can help guide better skincare practices and prevent acne from worsening. It's important to treat acne based on its type and severity to avoid long-term skin damage.

1.2 Main causes of acne (hormones, diet, lifestyle, environment)

Acne is a common skin condition that affects many people, especially during adolescence. Understanding the main causes can help in managing and preventing breakouts. **Here's a breakdown of the key factors:**

1. Hormones

Hormonal changes are one of the primary contributors to acne. During puberty, increased levels of androgens (male hormones present in both men and women) stimulate the sebaceous glands in the skin. This leads to increased oil production, which can clog pores and create an environment for bacteria to thrive. Hormonal fluctuations related to menstrual cycles, pregnancy, or conditions like polycystic ovary syndrome (PCOS) can also trigger acne flare-ups.

2. Diet

Diet plays a significant role in skin health. Certain foods may exacerbate acne. **For example:**

- **High glycemic index foods:** Foods that spike blood sugar levels, such as white bread, sugary snacks, and soft drinks, can lead to increased insulin levels. This, in turn, can trigger oil production and inflammation.
- **Dairy products:** Some studies suggest a link between dairy consumption and acne, possibly due to hormones present in milk.

- **Processed foods:** Diets high in processed foods and unhealthy fats may contribute to inflammation, which can worsen acne.

3. Lifestyle

Lifestyle choices significantly impact skin health. Factors to consider include:

- **Stress:** High stress levels can lead to increases in certain hormones that trigger oil production, leading to more breakouts.
- **Skincare routine:** Using harsh soaps or not cleansing the skin properly can irritate the skin and contribute to clogged pores. On the other hand, overly aggressive treatment can irritate the skin and exacerbate acne.
- **Physical activity:** Regular exercise can improve circulation and reduce stress. However, not showering after sweating can trap dirt and oil, leading to breakouts.

4. Environment

Environmental factors can also influence acne. Consider the following:

- **Humidity and pollution:** High humidity can increase oil production, while pollution can clog pores and irritate the skin.
- **Products and materials:** Certain cosmetics, hair products, and even some fabrics can contribute to acne. It's important to choose non-comedogenic products that won't block pores.

Acne is a complex condition influenced by various factors, including hormones, diet, lifestyle, and environmental elements. Understanding these causes can empower individuals to make informed choices that may help reduce breakouts and improve overall skin health. By adopting a balanced diet, managing stress, and choosing appropriate skincare products, it is possible to mitigate the effects of acne.

1.3 Why natural treatments work better for the skin.

Natural treatments often work better for the skin in clearing acne because they focus on healing from the inside out, using ingredients that are gentle and nourishing. **Here are several reasons why natural treatments can be more effective for acne:**

1. Less Irritation

Natural treatments usually contain fewer harsh chemicals, which means they are less likely to irritate or dry out the skin. Acne medications and treatments with strong chemicals can strip the skin of its natural oils, leading to dryness, redness, and even more breakouts. Natural ingredients like aloe vera or honey help soothe and calm the skin without causing irritation.

2. Balancing Oil Production

Many natural remedies help regulate the skin's oil production, which is one of the main causes of acne. For example, tea tree oil has natural antibacterial properties that can reduce the bacteria causing acne while balancing oil production. This reduces the risk of clogged pores, which often lead to breakouts.

3. Supporting Skin Healing

Natural treatments are packed with nutrients that support the skin's healing process. Ingredients like aloe vera, turmeric, and green tea have anti-inflammatory and antioxidant properties. These help the skin repair itself faster, reducing the appearance of acne scars and promoting an even skin tone.

4. Fewer Side Effects

Unlike many chemical-based treatments, natural remedies come with fewer side effects. Conventional acne treatments can cause peeling, burning, and sensitivity, especially for people with sensitive skin. Natural treatments are often gentler, reducing the likelihood of adverse reactions.

5. Promoting Long-Term Skin Health

Natural treatments don't just address acne but also improve overall skin health. They nourish the skin with vitamins and antioxidants, helping to maintain moisture, elasticity, and smoothness. This leads to healthier skin in the long term, preventing future breakouts.

6. Holistic Approach

Natural treatments often take a holistic approach, addressing not just the surface of the skin but also lifestyle factors like diet, stress, and sleep. For example, eating foods rich in omega-3 fatty acids, reducing sugar intake, and staying hydrated can improve skin health from the inside, preventing acne from reoccurring.

Natural treatments work better for the skin because they are gentler, support natural healing, and promote overall skin health without the harsh side effects of chemical-based acne treatments. They not only clear acne but also contribute to long-term skin wellness.

Chapter 2

Natural Skincare Routines for Clear Skin

2.1 Daily and weekly skincare routines

To naturally clear acne, a consistent daily and weekly skincare routine can help maintain clean, healthy skin without harsh chemicals. This routine uses simple, natural ingredients that are easy to find and gentle on the skin. **Here's a step-by-step guide:**

Daily Skincare Routine for Clear Skin

Morning Routine:

1. Cleanse

Ingredients:

Honey (raw, organic) or a gentle natural cleanser with tea tree oil.

Instructions:

Start by washing your face with lukewarm water. Apply a small amount of honey to damp skin and gently massage it in for about 30 seconds. Honey has antibacterial properties that help reduce acne-causing bacteria. Rinse off with lukewarm water and pat dry with a clean towel.

2. Tone

Ingredients:

Witch hazel or rose water.

Instructions:

Pour a little witch hazel or rose water on a cotton pad and gently wipe it across your face. These natural toners help balance your skin's pH and reduce excess oil, which can cause breakouts.

3. Moisturize

Ingredients:

Aloe vera gel or jojoba oil.

Instructions:

Apply a small amount of aloe vera gel or jojoba oil to your skin. Aloe vera helps soothe and heal, while jojoba oil mimics the skin's natural oils, keeping it moisturized without clogging pores.

4. Sun Protection

Ingredients:

Mineral sunscreen (zinc oxide or titanium dioxide).

Instructions:

Even if you're staying indoors, apply a natural sunscreen with at least SPF 30. Sunscreen protects your skin from UV rays, which can worsen acne and cause scarring.

Evening Routine:

1. Cleanse Again

Ingredients:

Oatmeal and water or a mild cleanser.

Instructions:

In the evening, wash your face again using a gentle cleanser. You can also use a mixture of finely ground oatmeal and water as a soothing, natural cleanser that won't irritate acne-prone skin.

2. Exfoliate (2-3 times a week)
Ingredients:

Baking soda (optional) or oatmeal.

Instructions:

Mix 1 tablespoon of baking soda with a little water to make a paste (or use ground oatmeal). Gently massage this mixture onto your skin for about 30 seconds. Avoid scrubbing too hard, as it can irritate acne. Rinse with cool water.

3. Spot Treatment (As needed)

Ingredients:

Tea tree oil or apple cider vinegar (diluted).

Instructions:

For active breakouts, apply a small dab of tea tree oil directly to the pimple using a cotton swab. Tea tree oil has natural antibacterial properties. If using apple cider vinegar, dilute it with water (1 part vinegar to 3 parts water) and apply with a cotton swab.

4. Moisturize

Ingredients:

Rosehip oil or aloe vera gel.

Instructions:

Apply a light layer of rosehip oil or aloe vera gel to help the skin repair itself while you sleep. Rosehip oil is rich in vitamins that promote skin healing, while aloe vera soothes and reduces inflammation.

Weekly Skincare Routine for Clear Skin

1. Deep Cleansing Mask (1-2 times a week):

Ingredients:

Bentonite clay or kaolin clay.

Water or apple cider vinegar.

Instructions:

Mix 1 tablespoon of clay with a small amount of water or apple cider vinegar to form a paste. Apply the paste evenly over your face and leave it on for 10-15 minutes until it dries. Clay helps draw out impurities and excess oil from the pores. Use lukewarm water to rinse, then carefully pat the skin dry.

2. Steam Treatment (Once a week):

Ingredients:

Hot water and optional essential oils (lavender, tea tree).

Instructions:

Boil water and pour it into a bowl. If desired, add a few drops of an essential oil like lavender or tea tree. Lean over the bowl with a towel over your head to trap the steam. Let the steam cleanse your pores for about 5-10 minutes. Afterward, splash your face with cool water to close your pores.

3. Hydrating Mask (Once a week):

Ingredients:

Avocado and honey.

Instructions:

Mash half an avocado and mix it with 1 tablespoon of honey. Apply the mixture to your face and let it sit for 15-20 minutes. Avocado provides deep hydration, while honey helps soothe and heal the skin. Rinse off with lukewarm water.

Additional Tips for Naturally Clear Skin

Stay Hydrated: Drink at least 8 glasses of water daily to keep your skin hydrated from the inside out.

Balanced Diet: Eat foods rich in antioxidants (like leafy greens, berries, and nuts) and omega-3 fatty acids (from fish or flaxseeds) to support skin health.

Manage Stress: Practice relaxation techniques like yoga or meditation, as stress can trigger acne flare-ups.

Get Enough Sleep: Aim for 7-9 hours of sleep each night to give your skin time to repair itself.

By following this daily and weekly skincare routine using natural ingredients, you can help keep acne at bay and maintain clear, healthy skin.

2.2 Skincare tips for different skin types (oily, dry, combination, sensitive).

1. Oily Skin

Oily skin tends to produce excess sebum, leading to shine, enlarged pores, and frequent breakouts. The goal is to balance oil production without over-drying the skin.

Cleanse twice a day: Use a gentle foaming or gel cleanser to remove dirt and oil. Avoid harsh cleansers that strip the skin, as they can cause more oil production.

Exfoliate regularly: Exfoliate 2-3 times a week with a mild exfoliant to clear away dead skin cells and prevent clogged pores.

Use oil-free moisturizers: Even oily skin needs moisture. Choose a lightweight, oil-free moisturizer to hydrate without clogging pores.

Apply mattifying products: Products with ingredients like salicylic acid or tea tree oil can help control shine and prevent acne.

Don't skip sunscreen: Use a non-comedogenic (won't clog pores) sunscreen daily to protect against sun damage without making your skin greasy.

2. Dry Skin

Dry skin lacks moisture, which can make it feel tight, flaky, and even rough. The focus here is to keep your skin hydrated and well-nourished.

Use a creamy cleanser: Look for hydrating cleansers that cleanse without stripping your skin of natural oils.

Moisturize immediately after washing: After cleansing, apply a rich, hydrating moisturizer while your skin is still damp to lock in moisture.

Avoid hot water: Hot water can strip your skin of its natural oils, making it drier. Opt for mildly warm water when cleansing your face for optimal results.

Choose thicker creams: Opt for thick, oil-based creams or balms that provide long-lasting hydration. Ingredients like shea butter, glycerin, and hyaluronic acid work well.

Exfoliate gently: Exfoliate once a week to remove dead skin cells, but use a gentle exfoliator to avoid further drying your skin.

3. Combination Skin

Combination skin has both oily and dry areas, often with an oily T-zone (forehead, nose, and chin) and dry cheeks. The key is to balance hydration and oil control.

Use a gentle cleanser: Look for a balanced cleanser that cleans without overly drying or making your skin oily.

Moisturize strategically: Use a lightweight, oil-free moisturizer on your T-zone and a richer cream on drier areas like your cheeks.

Spot-treat problem areas: If your T-zone gets oily or prone to breakouts, apply a mattifying or acne-fighting treatment just to those areas.

Exfoliate with care: Exfoliate once or twice a week, focusing on oily areas while being gentle on the drier parts.

Hydrating masks: Use hydrating masks on the drier parts of your face and clay-based masks on the oily areas for a balanced approach.

4. Sensitive Skin

Sensitive skin can be easily irritated by products and environmental factors. The focus is on gentle, soothing products to prevent flare-ups and discomfort.

Choose gentle, fragrance-free cleansers: Opt for cleansers labeled as hypoallergenic or made for sensitive skin, avoiding those with strong fragrances or harsh chemicals.

Moisturize with soothing ingredients: Look for moisturizers that contain calming ingredients like aloe vera, chamomile, or ceramides to strengthen your skin's barrier and reduce irritation.

Patch-test new products: Before using any new product, patch-test it on a small area of your skin to ensure it doesn't cause a reaction.

Use sunscreen carefully: Choose sunscreens that are formulated for sensitive skin, usually labeled as mineral-based with ingredients like zinc oxide or titanium dioxide.

Limit exfoliation: Exfoliate very gently and infrequently, about once a week, using mild exfoliants to avoid triggering irritation.

By understanding your skin type and using products that address its specific needs, you can maintain healthier, clearer, and more balanced skin.

2.3 Essential natural ingredients for clear skin.

When looking to clear acne naturally, certain essential natural ingredients have proven to be highly effective. These ingredients not only help reduce inflammation and kill bacteria but also promote overall skin health. **Here's a comprehensive list of essential natural ingredients for clear skin:**

1. Tea Tree Oil

Tea tree oil is one of the most popular natural remedies for acne. It has antibacterial properties that help fight acne-causing bacteria. Additionally, it reduces redness and inflammation, which can make breakouts less noticeable.

How to Use: Dilute a few drops of tea tree oil with a carrier oil (like coconut or jojoba oil) and apply it to the affected areas.

2. Aloe Vera

Aloe vera is well-known for its soothing and healing properties. It helps calm irritated skin, reduces inflammation, and promotes faster healing of acne lesions. Its moisturizing properties also prevent the skin from drying out.

How to Use: Apply fresh aloe vera gel directly to the skin, especially to inflamed or red areas. Leave it on for 20 minutes before rinsing.

3. Honey

Honey has natural antibacterial and anti-inflammatory properties. It helps cleanse the skin, reduce bacteria, and keep it hydrated. Honey also acts as a gentle exfoliant, removing dead skin cells that can clog pores.

How to Use: Apply a thin layer of raw honey to the face as a mask. Leave it on for 15-20 minutes and rinse with warm water.

4. Apple Cider Vinegar

Apple cider vinegar (ACV) helps balance the skin's pH levels, making it more difficult for acne-causing bacteria to thrive. It also has mild exfoliating properties, which help unclog pores and remove dead skin cells.

How to Use: Mix ACV with water (1:3 ratio) and use a cotton pad to apply it to your face after cleansing. Avoid using ACV undiluted, as it can irritate the skin.

5. Witch Hazel

Witch hazel is a natural astringent that tightens skin and reduces inflammation. It can help control oil production and soothe irritated, acne-prone skin.

How to Use: Apply witch hazel using a cotton ball after cleansing to tone the skin and reduce excess oil.

6. Green Tea

Green tea contains powerful antioxidants called catechins, which reduce inflammation and fight bacteria. Topical green tea can calm irritated skin and help prevent future breakouts.

How to Use: Brew green tea and allow it to cool. Use a cotton ball to apply it to your face or mix the cooled tea with other natural ingredients like honey for a mask.

7. Jojoba Oil

Although using oil on acne-prone skin may seem counterintuitive, jojoba oil is a lightweight, non-comedogenic oil that mimics the skin's natural oils. It helps balance sebum production and prevents pores from becoming clogged.

How to Use: Apply a few drops of jojoba oil directly to your skin after cleansing. It can be used as a moisturizer or a spot treatment.

8. Turmeric

Turmeric has strong anti-inflammatory and antimicrobial properties. It helps reduce redness, kill acne-causing bacteria, and improve overall skin tone.

How to Use: Mix turmeric with honey or yogurt to create a mask. Apply it to your face and leave it on for 15 minutes before rinsing.

9. Oatmeal

Oatmeal is soothing to the skin and helps absorb excess oil. It also has gentle exfoliating properties, which can help prevent clogged pores.

How to Use: Cook plain oatmeal and let it cool. Apply it as a mask and leave it on for 15-20 minutes before rinsing.

10. Lemon Juice

Lemon juice contains natural citric acid, which helps exfoliate the skin and unclog pores. It also has antibacterial properties and can reduce acne scars over time.

How to Use: Dilute lemon juice with water and apply it to your skin using a cotton ball. Be sure to rinse it off after 10 minutes, as it can be drying and may increase sun sensitivity.

Tips for Best Results:

Always do a patch test before applying any of these ingredients to your face, especially if you have sensitive skin.

Combine these ingredients with a healthy skincare routine that includes gentle cleansing and moisturizing.

Drink plenty of water and maintain a balanced diet rich in fruits and vegetables to support healthy skin from within.

By using these natural ingredients regularly, you can help clear your acne while keeping your skin healthy and radiant.

Chapter 3

DIY Acne-Fighting Remedies

3.1 Face masks for acne-prone skin.

Face masks for acne-prone skin can be a powerful way to soothe irritation, reduce breakouts, and balance oily skin. Creating DIY acne-fighting face masks at home allows you to control the ingredients, ensuring you're using natural and effective remedies that target the root causes of acne, such as excess oil, clogged pores, and inflammation. **Here's a clear and simple guide to a few effective DIY acne-fighting face masks:**

1. Honey and Cinnamon Mask

Honey has natural antibacterial properties, making it great for fighting acne-causing bacteria. Cinnamon is also antibacterial and can reduce inflammation, helping to soothe acne-prone skin.

Ingredients:

2 tablespoons of raw honey

1 teaspoon of cinnamon

Instructions:

1. Mix the honey and cinnamon into a smooth paste.

2. Apply it to your face, avoiding the eye area.

3. Leave it on for 10-15 minutes, then rinse off with warm water.

This mask helps to kill acne-causing bacteria and calm irritated skin.

2. Turmeric and Yogurt Mask

Turmeric is known for its anti-inflammatory and antimicrobial properties, making it a great choice for acne-prone skin. Yogurt contains lactic acid, which gently exfoliates dead skin cells, unclogs pores, and helps lighten acne scars.

Ingredients:

1 tablespoon of plain yogurt

1 teaspoon of turmeric powder

Instructions:

1. Mix the yogurt and turmeric into a paste.

2. Apply to your face and let it sit for 10-15 minutes.

3. Rinse thoroughly with lukewarm water.

This mask helps reduce redness and inflammation while gently exfoliating the skin.

3. Aloe Vera and Tea Tree Oil Mask

Aloe vera is soothing and helps reduce redness and inflammation, while tea tree oil is a powerful antibacterial that fights acne-causing bacteria.

Ingredients:

2 tablespoons of fresh aloe vera gel

2-3 drops of tea tree oil

Instructions:

1. Mix the aloe vera gel with tea tree oil.

2. Apply the mixture to your face, focusing on acne-prone areas.

3. Leave it on for 15-20 minutes before rinsing off.

This mask helps calm irritated skin and fight acne-causing bacteria.

4. Oatmeal and Honey Mask

Oatmeal is a gentle exfoliant that absorbs excess oil and removes dead skin cells, while honey's antibacterial properties help heal existing breakouts.

Ingredients:

2 tablespoons of cooked oatmeal (cooled)

1 tablespoon of honey

Instructions:

1. Mix the oatmeal and honey into a thick paste.

2. Apply the mask to your face and leave it on for 15-20 minutes.

3. Rinse off with warm water, gently massaging your skin in circular motions.

This mask is excellent for both soothing irritated skin and gently removing impurities.

5. Green Tea and Clay Mask

Green tea contains antioxidants that help reduce inflammation and fight free radicals, while clay absorbs excess oil and detoxifies the skin.

Ingredients:

1 tablespoon of green tea (brewed and cooled)

1 tablespoon of bentonite or kaolin clay

Instructions:

1. Mix the green tea with the clay to form a smooth paste.

2. Apply to your face and leave it on until the mask dries (about 10-15 minutes).

3. Rinse with lukewarm water and pat your skin dry.

This mask is great for deep cleaning the pores and controlling oil production.

General Tips for Using Face Masks:

Frequency: Use these masks 1-2 times per week for the best results. Overuse can dry out the skin, which may lead to more oil production and breakouts.

Spot Test: Always do a patch test before applying a new mask to your face, especially if you have sensitive skin.

Hydrate Afterward: After rinsing off the mask, follow up with a gentle moisturizer to keep your skin hydrated and balanced.

By using simple, natural ingredients, you can create effective DIY face masks that help fight acne, reduce inflammation, and promote clearer, healthier skin.

3.2 Simple recipes for natural toners and spot treatments.

Natural toners and spot treatments can be made easily at home with ingredients that are gentle on the skin yet effective in managing acne. These DIY solutions help balance the skin, reduce inflammation, and clear up acne over time. **Here are a few simple recipes:**

1. Apple Cider Vinegar Toner

Apple cider vinegar helps balance the skin's pH and has antibacterial properties to fight acne.

Ingredients:

1 part raw, unfiltered apple cider vinegar

2 parts water (for sensitive skin, use 3-4 parts water)

Instructions:

Mix the apple cider vinegar and water in a small bottle.

After washing your face, apply the mixture with a cotton ball or pad.

Let it dry and then follow up with your moisturizer.

2. Green Tea Toner

Green tea is rich in antioxidants and helps reduce inflammation and sebum production, making it great for acne-prone skin.

Ingredients:

1 green tea bag

1 cup boiling water

Instructions:

Steep the green tea bag in boiling water for 5-10 minutes.

Allow the tea to cool completely.

Transfer it to a spray bottle or jar and use it as a toner after cleansing your face. Store in the fridge for up to a week.

3. Witch Hazel and Aloe Vera Spot Treatment

Witch hazel is a natural astringent, and aloe vera soothes the skin while reducing redness and inflammation.

Ingredients:

2 tablespoons witch hazel

1 tablespoon aloe vera gel

Instructions:

Combine the witch hazel with the aloe vera gel.

Apply the mixture to acne spots using a cotton swab or clean fingers.

Let it sit for a few minutes before applying your regular moisturizer.

DIY Acne-Fighting Remedies

These acne-fighting remedies use simple, natural ingredients that you likely already have at home. They help clear acne, reduce inflammation, and prevent future breakouts.

1. Honey and Cinnamon Spot Treatment

Honey has antibacterial properties, and cinnamon can help reduce inflammation.

Ingredients:

1 teaspoon raw honey

½ teaspoon cinnamon powder

Instructions:

Mix the honey and cinnamon to form a paste.

Apply the paste to acne spots and leave it on for 10-15 minutes.

Rinse off with warm water and pat dry.

2. Tea Tree Oil Spot Treatment

Tea tree oil is a powerful antibacterial agent that can help reduce acne quickly.

Ingredients:

1-2 drops tea tree oil

1 teaspoon carrier oil (like jojoba or coconut oil)

Instructions:

Dilute the tea tree oil with the carrier oil to avoid skin irritation.

Using a cotton swab, apply the mixture directly to acne spots.

Leave it on overnight and rinse off in the morning.

3. Oatmeal and Honey Face Mask

Oatmeal is soothing and can help reduce inflammation, while honey's antibacterial properties help fight acne.

Ingredients:

1 tablespoon oatmeal (ground)

1 tablespoon honey

A little water if needed

Instructions:

Mix the ground oatmeal and honey to form a paste.

Apply it to your face and leave it on for 15-20 minutes.

Rinse with warm water, massaging the skin gently in circular motions.

4. Turmeric and Yogurt Mask

Turmeric has anti-inflammatory and antibacterial properties, while yogurt contains lactic acid, which can gently exfoliate the skin.

Ingredients:

1 teaspoon turmeric powder

2 tablespoons plain yogurt

Instructions:

Mix the turmeric and yogurt to create a smooth paste.

Apply the mask to your face and leave it on for 10-15 minutes.

Rinse thoroughly with warm water.

By using these natural, DIY recipes, you can help manage acne in a gentle yet effective way, without exposing your skin to harsh chemicals. Regular use of these treatments can lead to clearer, healthier skin.

3.3 How to exfoliate acne-prone skin gently.
Exfoliating acne-prone skin requires a delicate approach to avoid irritation, which can lead to more breakouts. The goal is to remove dead skin cells, unclog pores, and promote skin renewal without causing redness or inflammation. **Here's how to exfoliate acne-prone skin gently:**

1. Choose the Right Exfoliant

It's crucial to use a gentle exfoliant, especially if you have sensitive skin or active acne. Avoid harsh scrubs with large, rough particles, as they can damage the skin. Instead, opt for chemical exfoliants with salicylic acid or glycolic acid, which work by dissolving dead skin cells without the need for scrubbing. These ingredients are especially good for acne-prone skin because they penetrate the pores and help to prevent future breakouts.

2. Limit Exfoliation Frequency

Over-exfoliating can strip your skin of its natural oils, leading to dryness and irritation, which can trigger more acne. Start by exfoliating only 1-2 times per week. If your skin tolerates it well, you can gradually increase the frequency, but always monitor how your skin reacts.

3. Use Gentle Tools

If you prefer physical exfoliation, use a soft washcloth or a silicone cleansing brush. These tools are less abrasive than grainy scrubs and still help remove impurities from the skin. Be sure to apply light pressure to avoid irritation.

4. Moisturize After Exfoliating

Exfoliation can leave your skin feeling dry, especially if you have acne-prone skin. After exfoliating, it's essential to apply a light, non-comedogenic moisturizer to help soothe and hydrate your skin. Look for ingredients like hyaluronic acid or aloe vera, which are known for their hydrating and calming properties.

DIY Acne-Fighting Remedies

In addition to gentle exfoliation, there are a few natural remedies you can try to help fight acne and keep your skin clear. These remedies use simple ingredients you might already have at home:

1. Honey and Cinnamon Mask

Honey is a natural humectant, meaning it draws moisture into the skin, while cinnamon has anti-inflammatory and antibacterial properties. Together, they can help reduce acne and calm irritated skin.

How to Use:

Mix 2 tablespoons of honey with 1 teaspoon of cinnamon.

Apply the mixture to your face and leave it on for 10-15 minutes before rinsing off with warm water.

2. Tea Tree Oil Spot Treatment

Tea tree oil is known for its antibacterial and anti-inflammatory properties, making it an effective natural treatment for acne.

How to Use:

Dilute 1-2 drops of tea tree oil with a carrier oil (like jojoba or coconut oil).

Apply the mixture directly to acne spots using a cotton swab.

Let it sit overnight and wash it off in the morning.

3. Aloe Vera and Green Tea Toner

Aloe vera is soothing and hydrating, while green tea contains antioxidants that can help reduce inflammation and redness. Together, they make a great toner for acne-prone skin.

How to Use:

Brew a cup of green tea and let it cool.

Mix the green tea with 1 tablespoon of aloe vera gel.

Apply it to your skin using a cotton pad after cleansing, and let it dry naturally.

4. Oatmeal and Yogurt Exfoliating Mask

Oatmeal is gentle and soothing, making it a great option for sensitive or acne-prone skin. Yogurt contains lactic acid, a mild exfoliant that helps brighten the skin and remove dead cells.

How to Use:

Mix 2 tablespoons of plain yogurt with 1 tablespoon of ground oatmeal.

Apply the mixture to your face, gently massaging it in circular motions.

Leave it on for 10-15 minutes before rinsing off with lukewarm water.

Tips for Best Results

Patch Test First: Always do a patch test on a small area of skin to make sure you don't have an allergic reaction to any DIY remedy.

Stay Consistent: Consistency is key when it comes to skincare. Stick with your routine and give it time—most skincare products take a few weeks to show results.

Be Gentle: Avoid scrubbing or applying too much pressure, especially when exfoliating. Gentle motions will give you the best results without damaging your skin.

By combining gentle exfoliation with these acne-fighting remedies, you can create a balanced skincare routine that keeps your skin clear and healthy without causing irritation.

Chapter 4

Healing Acne Scars Naturally

4.1 Types of acne scars (hyperpigmentation, pitted scars).

Acne scars come in different forms and can leave lasting marks on the skin, even after the breakouts have cleared. These scars generally fall into two main types: **hyperpigmentation** and **pitted** scars. Understanding the differences between them can help guide treatment options.

1. Hyperpigmentation

Hyperpigmentation refers to the dark spots or areas of discoloration that remain on the skin after acne heals. It's not technically a scar but rather a change in skin color due to inflammation. This type of scarring occurs when the skin produces excess melanin, the pigment responsible for skin color, as part of the healing process. The spots can range from red, pink, brown, or even purple, depending on your skin tone.

Causes: Hyperpigmentation is often caused by picking or squeezing pimples, as well as by sun exposure during the healing process.

Treatment: This type of scarring can fade over time, but treatments such as topical creams containing ingredients like vitamin C, retinoids, or niacinamide can help speed up the process. Regular sunscreen use is crucial to prevent further darkening of these spots.

2. Pitted Scars

Pitted scars, also called atrophic scars, are deeper than hyperpigmentation and result from more severe acne, like cystic acne. These scars form when the skin tissue is damaged and doesn't heal properly, leading to depressions or indents in the skin. **There are different kinds of pitted scars, including:**

Ice pick scars: These are deep and narrow scars that look like tiny holes punctured into the skin. They are difficult to treat because of their depth.

Boxcar scars: These are wider and more rectangular in shape, with sharp edges. They can be shallow or deep, depending on how much skin tissue was lost.

Rolling scars: These scars create a wave-like texture on the skin, with broad depressions and sloped edges. They are caused by bands of scar tissue under the skin, pulling it downwards.

Causes: Pitted scars form when there is a loss of skin tissue during the healing process of more severe acne. Inflammation destroys collagen, and the skin is unable to regenerate fully, resulting in uneven texture.

Treatment: Pitted scars are more challenging to treat and often require professional procedures such as microneedling, laser therapy, chemical peels, or fillers. These treatments work to stimulate collagen production and smooth the skin's surface.

Both hyperpigmentation and pitted scars are common after-effects of acne, but they differ significantly in appearance and treatment needs. Hyperpigmentation is primarily a discoloration that can fade with time and proper skincare, while pitted scars involve changes to the skin's texture and often require more intensive treatments.

4.2 Natural remedies to fade scars (essential oils, gentle exfoliation).

Acne scars can be stubborn, but natural remedies using essential oils and gentle exfoliation can help fade them over time. These methods promote healing and improve the texture of your skin without harsh chemicals.

1. Essential Oils for Fading Scars

Essential oils are known for their skin-healing properties. They help to lighten scars, promote cell regeneration, and reduce inflammation. Here are some of the most effective oils for fading acne scars:

a. Tea Tree Oil

Properties: Tea tree oil has powerful anti-inflammatory and antimicrobial properties that can reduce the appearance of scars.

Instructions:

Mix 2-3 drops of tea tree oil with 1 teaspoon of a carrier oil (such as coconut or jojoba oil).

Gently massage the mixture onto your scars twice daily.

Do not apply undiluted tea tree oil directly to the skin, as it may cause irritation.

b. Rosehip Oil

Properties: Rosehip oil is rich in vitamins A and C, which boost collagen production and improve skin texture.

Instructions:

Apply a few drops of rosehip oil directly onto the scarred areas.

Massage it gently in a circular motion for a few minutes.

Use it before bed and leave it on overnight.

c. Lavender Oil

Properties: Lavender oil helps to regenerate skin cells and has calming effects that promote healing.

Instructions:

Combine 4-5 drops of lavender oil with 1 teaspoon of a carrier oil.

Apply the mixture to your scars every evening.

Allow it to absorb into the skin for at least 20 minutes before rinsing or leaving it overnight.

2. Gentle Exfoliation for the Effective Removal of Dead Skin Cells

Exfoliating your skin helps to remove dead skin cells and encourages new skin growth. However, it's essential to use gentle ingredients to avoid irritation, especially for acne scars.

a. Oatmeal and Honey Exfoliating Mask

Properties: Oatmeal soothes and gently exfoliates, while honey has antibacterial and healing properties.

Ingredients:

2 tablespoons of ground oatmeal

1 tablespoon of honey

1 tablespoon of water (or yogurt for added moisture)

Instructions:

Combine the ingredients until a smooth paste is achieved.

Gently apply the mask to your face, concentrating on the areas with scarring.

Massage gently for 2-3 minutes in circular motions, then leave it on for another 10-15 minutes.

Rinse with warm water. Use 2-3 times per week.

b. Sugar and Olive Oil Scrub

Properties: Sugar acts as a natural exfoliant, while olive oil moisturizes and nourishes the skin.

Ingredients:

1 tablespoon of sugar (preferably brown sugar for its gentleness)

1 tablespoon of olive oil

Instructions:

Mix the sugar and olive oil together to form a scrub.

Gently rub the scrub onto the scarred areas for about 2-3 minutes.

Rinse off with warm water. Use once or twice a week for best results.

3. Natural Moisturizers to Support Healing

Keeping the skin moisturized is essential for fading scars, as dryness can hinder the healing process.

a. Aloe Vera Gel

Properties: Aloe vera is soothing, promotes skin regeneration, and helps lighten scars over time.

Instructions:

Apply pure aloe vera gel (from a store or directly from the plant) onto the affected areas.

Leave it on for 30 minutes, then rinse with lukewarm water.

Repeat daily for best results.

b. Coconut Oil

Properties: Coconut oil is rich in antioxidants and vitamins that help repair damaged skin and reduce scarring.

Instructions:

Warm up a small amount of coconut oil between your fingers.

Massage it into the scars for a few minutes, allowing it to absorb fully.

You can leave it on overnight for deeper moisturization.

Consistency is key when using natural remedies to fade scars. It may take weeks or even months to see significant improvements, but using these gentle and nourishing methods will help heal your skin naturally without irritation. Be patient, and remember that every skin type responds differently.

4.3 Long-term healing and prevention of scars.

Long-term healing and prevention of scars, especially from acne, requires patience and a holistic approach. When treating acne scars naturally, it's important to focus on three main areas: skin repair, scar prevention, and maintenance.

1. Skin Repair

Your skin needs to heal from the inside out, and you can support this by providing the right nutrients. A diet rich in vitamins A, C, and E is essential, as these vitamins help repair skin tissue. Zinc and omega-3 fatty acids also promote healing and reduce inflammation. Hydration is key—drink plenty of water to keep your skin moisturized and support the natural healing process.

2. Natural Remedies for Healing Scars

There are several natural remedies that can help fade acne scars over time:

Aloe Vera: Aloe vera gel helps regenerate skin tissue. Applying fresh aloe vera to scars daily can soothe the skin and help it heal faster.

Rosehip Oil: Rich in fatty acids and vitamin A, rosehip oil has been shown to reduce the appearance of scars when applied consistently.

Honey: Honey has natural healing properties and can be applied to scars to help soften them over time. It also helps keep the skin moisturized, which is crucial for scar healing.

Lemon Juice: Although it's a bit stronger, lemon juice can help lighten scars thanks to its natural bleaching properties. However, it should be used sparingly, and always with sunscreen afterward, as it can make the skin more sensitive to sunlight.

Coconut Oil: Coconut oil is full of antioxidants and vitamin E, which help repair skin and reduce scars. Gently massaging it into scarred areas can improve texture and appearance over time.

3. Preventing Future Scarring

The best way to prevent acne scars is to treat acne early and avoid aggravating the skin. Never pick or squeeze pimples, as this damages the skin and increases the risk of scars. **You should also:**

Moisturize Regularly: Keeping your skin hydrated helps it heal and remain flexible, which can prevent scarring.

Use Sunscreen: Sun exposure can darken scars and make them more noticeable. Wearing sunscreen daily, even on cloudy days, will protect your skin and help scars fade faster.

Exfoliate Gently: Gentle exfoliation with a natural scrub or a mild chemical exfoliant like lactic acid can remove dead skin cells, helping new, healthy skin emerge. Be careful not to over-exfoliate, as this can irritate the skin and slow healing.

4. Consistency is Key

Natural scar treatment requires consistency. It can take weeks or even months to see noticeable improvement, so it's important to be patient and stick with your routine. Regular application of natural oils, masks, and moisturizing treatments will yield long-term results.

5. Lifestyle Habits for Prevention

In addition to topical treatments, a healthy lifestyle supports long-term skin health. Ensure you get enough sleep, manage stress, and maintain a balanced diet. Stress can lead to breakouts, and breakouts lead to scars, so managing both can prevent future issues.

6. Patience in Healing

Remember that healing acne scars naturally is a gradual process. Avoid quick-fix solutions, as they can sometimes do more harm than good. By nurturing your skin over time and providing it with the right care, you can achieve smoother, healthier skin and prevent future scars from forming.

The key to success is a consistent, natural skincare routine, combined with healthy lifestyle habits. This will not only help fade existing scars but also prevent new ones from forming, leading to long-term skin health.

Chapter 5

Diet and Acne: Eating for Clear Skin

5.1 The gut-skin connection: How your diet affects your skin.

The connection between the gut and skin is strong, and what you eat can significantly affect the health of your skin. This relationship is often referred to as the "gut-skin connection." Your digestive system and skin are linked through a balance of bacteria, inflammation levels, and nutrient absorption. When the gut is healthy, it helps reduce inflammation, supports proper nutrient absorption, and keeps your skin clear. On the other hand, an unhealthy gut can lead to skin issues like acne, dryness, or irritation.

Diet and Acne: Understanding the Link

Acne, one of the most common skin problems, can often be triggered by diet. While it's not the sole cause of acne, certain foods can make it worse by causing inflammation or hormonal imbalances. For example, foods high in sugar and processed carbs, like sweets, sodas, or white bread, spike blood sugar levels. This triggers the body to produce more insulin, which can lead to excess oil production and clogged pores, creating an environment for acne to thrive.

Similarly, dairy products have been linked to acne in some people. Milk, especially low-fat varieties, can affect hormone levels, which may increase the likelihood of breakouts. While not everyone will be affected the same way, keeping an eye on how your skin reacts to certain foods can help you identify potential triggers.

Eating for Clear Skin: What to Include in Your Diet

If you want to support clear, healthy skin, a balanced diet rich in whole, unprocessed foods is key. **Here are some skin-friendly food groups to focus on:**

1. Antioxidant-rich fruits and vegetables: Foods like berries, leafy greens, carrots, and tomatoes are packed with vitamins like A, C, and E. These antioxidants help fight off damage from free radicals, which can cause inflammation and contribute to skin aging and breakouts.

2. Healthy fats: Omega-3 fatty acids, found in foods like salmon, walnuts, and flaxseeds, are great for reducing inflammation in the body, which can help prevent acne and other skin conditions. Healthy fats also support the skin's natural moisture barrier, keeping it hydrated and supple.

3. Probiotic-rich foods: Fermented foods like yogurt, kefir, sauerkraut, and kimchi contain beneficial bacteria that help maintain a healthy gut. A well-balanced gut microbiome reduces inflammation and can improve overall skin health.

4. Zinc-rich foods: Zinc is a mineral that plays an important role in healing the skin and reducing inflammation. Foods like pumpkin seeds, chickpeas, and beef are good sources of zinc and can help prevent acne.

5. Hydrating foods: Water-rich foods like cucumbers, watermelon, and celery can help keep your skin hydrated from the inside out, reducing the risk of dryness and irritation.

Foods to Limit for Clear Skin

To support clearer skin, it's also helpful to limit certain foods that may trigger acne or other skin issues:

Sugary foods and drinks: As mentioned earlier, high-sugar foods can spike insulin levels, leading to inflammation and acne.

Processed carbs: White bread, pasta, and pastries can have a similar effect to sugar, increasing the risk of breakouts.

Dairy products: While not everyone is affected by dairy, some people may experience skin issues due to hormonal changes triggered by milk, cheese, or yogurt.

Fried and greasy foods: High levels of unhealthy fats found in fried foods can clog pores and contribute to acne.

Your diet has a powerful impact on your skin. By understanding the gut-skin connection, you can make informed choices about what you eat to support clear, healthy skin. Focusing on whole foods rich in antioxidants, healthy fats, and probiotics while limiting sugar and processed carbs can go a long way in preventing acne and promoting a glowing complexion. Remember, everyone's body is different, so paying attention to how your skin reacts to certain foods can help you build a diet that works best for your unique skin needs.

5.2 Foods to avoid that trigger acne.

To manage acne, it's important to avoid certain foods that can trigger breakouts or worsen the condition. **Here's a comprehensive guide to foods you should be careful about:**

1. Sugary Foods and Drinks

Foods and drinks high in sugar can cause spikes in blood sugar levels. When your blood sugar rises, your body releases insulin, which can increase oil production in your skin, leading to clogged pores and acne. **Examples include:**

Candy, cakes, and pastries

Sugary cereals

Sodas and sweetened beverages

Ice cream

2. Refined Carbohydrates

Refined carbs, like white bread, pasta, and processed snacks, break down quickly into sugar in your body, leading to increased insulin levels. This spike in insulin may contribute to acne. **Examples include:**

White bread and pasta

White rice

Chips, crackers, and other processed snacks

3. Dairy Products

Some studies suggest that dairy products, especially milk, may increase the risk of acne. This could be due to the hormones found in milk that can influence your skin's oil production. If you're prone to acne, **try reducing or avoiding:**

Milk (especially skim milk)

Cheese

Yogurt

Ice cream

4. Fast Food and Greasy Foods

Greasy, fast foods are typically high in unhealthy fats and refined carbs, which can lead to inflammation in the body. This inflammation can aggravate acne. **Common offenders include:**

Burgers, fries, and fried chicken

Pizza

Processed snack foods

5. Chocolate

Some people report that eating chocolate, especially milk chocolate, worsens their acne. Chocolate often contains sugar and dairy, which can both contribute to acne flare-ups. Opt for dark chocolate with low sugar content if you want a healthier alternative.

6. Foods High in Omega-6 Fats

Diets rich in omega-6 fats can promote inflammation, which may worsen acne. These fats are found in many processed foods and vegetable oils. **Try to limit:**

Corn oil, soybean oil, and sunflower oil

Processed snacks and fried foods

7. Whey Protein

Whey protein, a common supplement for building muscle, has been linked to acne, especially in teenagers and young adults. Whey protein can increase insulin levels, contributing to acne. If you use protein powders, consider switching to plant-based options.

8. Spicy Foods

Spicy foods can increase inflammation and heat in the body, which may trigger acne for some people. While spicy foods are not a universal acne trigger, it's best to monitor how your skin reacts if you consume them regularly.

By avoiding or limiting these foods, you may see an improvement in your acne. However, each person's skin reacts differently, so it's important to pay attention to how specific foods affect you. Consider keeping a food diary to track any links between your diet and acne flare-ups.

5.3 Acne-fighting superfoods and their benefits.

Acne-fighting superfoods are natural foods that can help reduce and prevent acne by promoting healthy skin. These foods are rich in vitamins, minerals, antioxidants, and other nutrients that support skin health and reduce inflammation, which is a major cause of acne. Including these superfoods in your diet can give your body the tools it needs to fight breakouts from the inside out.

1. Leafy Greens

Leafy greens like spinach, kale, and arugula are packed with vitamins A, C, and E. These vitamins help protect the skin from damage and support its ability to heal. Vitamin A is known to regulate skin cell production and reduce the risk of clogged pores, a common cause of acne. Vitamin C boosts collagen production, improving skin elasticity and repairing damage. Leafy greens also have a high water content, which helps keep your skin hydrated.

2. Fatty Fish

Fatty fish such as salmon, mackerel, and sardines are rich in omega-3 fatty acids. These healthy fats are anti-inflammatory, meaning they can reduce the redness and swelling associated with acne. Omega-3s also help maintain the skin's moisture barrier, preventing it from drying out. This balance of oils helps control the production of sebum, the oily substance that can clog pores and lead to breakouts.

3. Berries

Berries, including blueberries, strawberries, and raspberries, are full of antioxidants like vitamin C. Antioxidants help neutralize free radicals, unstable molecules that damage skin cells and trigger inflammation, which can worsen acne. The high vitamin C content also helps repair skin and reduce the appearance of acne scars.

4. **Nuts and Seeds**

Nuts and seeds, especially walnuts, almonds, chia seeds, and flaxseeds, are great sources of zinc, selenium, and omega-3 fatty acids. Zinc is essential for regulating oil production and can help reduce the severity of acne. Selenium is a powerful antioxidant that protects the skin from damage and helps it stay clear. Adding these to your diet can also promote overall skin health and give it a natural glow.

5. Sweet Potatoes

Sweet potatoes are high in beta-carotene, which the body converts into vitamin A. This nutrient helps prevent the overproduction of skin cells that can clog pores. Beta-carotene also protects the skin from sun damage, which can worsen acne or cause hyperpigmentation. Sweet potatoes are also a good source of fiber, which aids digestion and helps the body flush out toxins, contributing to clearer skin.

6. Green Tea

Green tea is rich in antioxidants, particularly catechins, which have anti-inflammatory and antibacterial properties. Drinking green tea regularly can help reduce the severity of acne by lowering the production of sebum and killing acne-causing bacteria. It also helps soothe irritated skin and reduce redness.

7. Probiotic-rich Foods

Foods like yogurt, kefir, sauerkraut, and kimchi contain probiotics, which are beneficial bacteria that improve gut health. A healthy gut is closely linked to clear skin, as digestive issues can lead to inflammation and acne. Probiotics help balance the gut microbiome, reduce inflammation, and promote a healthy immune system, all of which can result in fewer breakouts.

8. Avocados

Avocados are rich in vitamin E, an antioxidant that protects the skin from damage and helps it retain moisture. They also contain healthy fats that support skin hydration and reduce inflammation. Avocados can help improve the overall texture of the skin, making it softer and more resilient to breakouts.

9. Whole Grains

Whole grains like oats, quinoa, and brown rice are high in fiber and low on the glycemic index, meaning they don't cause a spike in blood sugar levels. High blood sugar can lead to increased insulin levels, which can trigger the production of hormones that cause acne. Eating whole grains helps keep your blood sugar stable, reducing the likelihood of acne flare-ups.

10. Carrots

Carrots are another great source of beta-carotene, which supports healthy skin and helps prevent clogged pores. Their high vitamin A content also aids in reducing inflammation and healing acne lesions. Eating carrots regularly can improve skin tone and help prevent new acne from forming.

Benefits of Including Acne-Fighting Superfoods:

Reduces inflammation: Many of these foods help calm the skin, preventing the redness and swelling that often accompanies acne.

Controls oil production: Superfoods rich in healthy fats and certain vitamins can help regulate sebum production, keeping pores clear.

Promotes skin healing: Foods high in antioxidants, vitamins, and minerals boost the skin's ability to repair itself, reducing the appearance of scars and preventing new breakouts.

Supports overall health: A diet rich in superfoods not only improves skin health but also boosts overall well-being, as these foods are packed with essential nutrients.

Incorporating these superfoods into your daily meals can help keep acne under control, leading to clearer, healthier skin. The key is consistency, as long-term changes in diet have the best impact on skin health.

Chapter 6

Daily Habits for Preventing Acne

6.1 The importance of hydration and its effect on skin.

Hydration is a key factor in maintaining healthy skin, and its importance cannot be overstated, especially when it comes to preventing acne. The skin is the largest organ in the body, and like any organ, it needs water to function properly. When you are properly hydrated, your skin can stay soft, smooth, and resilient, which plays a significant role in preventing acne.

How Hydration Affects the Skin

1. Balances Oil Production: One of the main benefits of staying hydrated is that it helps balance the skin's natural oil production. When your skin is well-hydrated, it doesn't feel the need to produce excess oil. Excess oil can clog pores, leading to breakouts. By drinking enough water, you help your skin maintain a proper oil balance, reducing the risk of clogged pores and acne.

2. Flushes Out Toxins: Hydration helps the body naturally flush out toxins. When you don't drink enough water, these toxins can accumulate and show up on your skin in the form of pimples and other blemishes. Drinking water helps your body expel these harmful substances, leading to clearer skin.

3. Improves Skin Cell Function: Water is essential for every cell in the body, including skin cells. When your skin is hydrated, its cells can function properly, heal faster, and renew themselves more efficiently. This helps keep your skin clear, healthy, and less prone to acne.

4. Prevents Dryness: Dry skin can be a major contributor to acne, especially if your skin tries to compensate by producing more oil. Hydrated skin stays moisturized naturally, which helps keep your skin's barrier strong and protected against irritants that can cause acne.

5. Promotes Elasticity and Healing: Well-hydrated skin retains its elasticity better and heals faster. This means that when breakouts do occur, your skin can recover more quickly, and you're less likely to experience long-term scarring or damage.

Staying hydrated is a simple yet powerful way to prevent acne and keep your skin healthy. By maintaining proper hydration, you support your skin's natural functions, promote healing, and prevent the buildup of toxins and oil that can lead to breakouts. Making hydration a daily habit can lead to clearer, smoother skin over time.

6.2 How stress affects acne and natural stress-reduction techniques.

Stress can significantly impact acne by triggering various physical responses in the body. When you're stressed, your body produces more cortisol, a hormone that can increase oil production in the skin. This excess oil can clog pores, leading to breakouts. Stress also weakens the immune system, making it harder for the body to fight off acne-causing bacteria. Inflammation caused by stress can worsen existing acne, making pimples more swollen and painful.

Stress can also lead to habits like touching your face or picking at acne, which can spread bacteria and make the problem worse. Emotional stress disrupts the balance of hormones in the body, particularly in teenagers and adults, which can further contribute to acne flare-ups.

Natural Stress-Reduction Techniques

1. Deep Breathing: Taking slow, deep breaths helps calm the nervous system. Deep breathing reduces cortisol levels, helping the body relax. Try practicing slow breathing exercises for a few minutes each day or whenever you're feeling stressed.

2. Mindfulness Meditation: Mindfulness involves focusing on the present moment and letting go of anxious thoughts. Regular meditation can help reduce stress, lower inflammation, and improve overall mental well-being, which in turn can reduce acne flare-ups.

3. Exercise: Physical activity helps reduce stress by releasing endorphins, which are chemicals that improve mood. Exercise also improves circulation, helping to nourish the skin and flush out toxins. Aim for regular movement, like walking, yoga, or any activity you enjoy.

4. Sleep: Getting enough quality sleep is crucial for stress management and skin health. During sleep, the body repairs and rejuvenates itself, including the skin. Lack of sleep increases stress, which can worsen acne. Aim for 7-9 hours of sleep each night.

5. Healthy Diet: Eating a balanced diet rich in fruits, vegetables, whole grains, and lean proteins can reduce inflammation and stress. Avoid sugary, processed foods, as they can contribute to acne and increase stress levels. Drinking plenty of water also helps keep the skin hydrated and healthy.

6. Journaling: Writing down your thoughts and feelings can help you process stress. It allows you to release pent-up emotions and reflect on what might be causing your stress, which can prevent it from affecting your skin.

7. Spending Time in Nature: Being outdoors and connecting with nature is a simple yet powerful way to reduce stress. Fresh air and natural surroundings can have a calming effect, lowering cortisol levels and helping you relax.

8. Social Support: Connecting with friends, family, or support groups can help you feel less alone and reduce stress. Talking about your worries can lighten the emotional load and give you a sense of relief.

By managing stress with these natural techniques, you can help prevent and reduce acne flare-ups, leading to healthier, clearer skin.

6.3 How sleep quality impacts skin health.
Sleep quality plays a vital role in keeping your skin healthy and clear of acne. When you don't get enough sleep or your sleep is poor, your body doesn't have enough time to repair and rejuvenate itself. This affects your skin's ability to heal and can make acne worse. **Here's how sleep quality impacts skin health, especially when it comes to clearing acne naturally:**

1. Hormonal Balance

Good sleep helps regulate hormones like cortisol, which is a stress hormone. High levels of cortisol can lead to increased oil production in the skin, which clogs pores and causes acne.

When you sleep well, your cortisol levels stay balanced, reducing the chance of breakouts.

2. Skin Repair and Regeneration

During sleep, your skin goes into repair mode. Cells regenerate, and your body produces new collagen, which helps keep your skin firm and clear. If you don't get enough sleep, your skin has less time to repair itself, which can slow the healing of acne and make scars more noticeable.

3. Reduced Inflammation

A good night's sleep reduces inflammation in your body. Inflammation is a major factor in the development of acne, making pimples red, swollen, and painful. Lack of sleep increases inflammation, making acne worse and preventing the skin from healing properly.

4. Immune System Support

Your immune system works to fight off bacteria and infections while you sleep. Acne can sometimes be caused by bacteria getting trapped in your pores. When you sleep poorly, your immune system becomes weaker, and it can't fight off these bacteria as effectively, leading to more acne breakouts.

5. Balanced Oil Production

When you sleep well, your skin's oil production stays balanced. However, lack of sleep causes your body to produce more oil, which clogs pores and leads to acne. A healthy sleep pattern can naturally help your skin maintain the right amount of moisture without becoming too oily.

6. Detoxification

While you sleep, your body detoxifies itself, flushing out harmful toxins. These toxins can affect your skin's health and lead to acne. When you don't get enough rest, the detoxification process is slowed down, and toxins can build up, leading to dull skin and more frequent breakouts.

How to Improve Sleep for Better Skin:

Stick to a consistent sleep schedule to help your body develop a natural rhythm.

Avoid caffeine and heavy meals before bed as they can interfere with sleep quality.

Create a relaxing bedtime routine, such as dimming lights or reading, to signal to your body that it's time to rest.

Limit screen time before bed since the blue light from devices can disrupt your sleep cycle.

Keep your sleep environment comfortable by adjusting room temperature and ensuring your bed is cozy.

By focusing on improving sleep quality, your body can naturally heal and maintain healthy skin, reducing the frequency and severity of acne breakouts.

Chapter 7

Long-Term Skincare Maintenance

7.1 How to track your skin's progress and adjust your regimen.

Tracking your skin's progress when using natural remedies for acne is essential for adjusting your regimen and achieving the best results. **Here's a comprehensive, clear guide on how to do this effectively:**

1. Keep a Skin Journal

Start by keeping a daily or weekly journal to record your skin's condition. Write down key observations, **such as:**

New breakouts

Redness or inflammation

Improvements, such as clearer skin or reduced pimples

Any changes in skin texture or dryness

What products or remedies you used that day

This will help you identify patterns and determine what's working for your skin over time.

2. Take Regular Photos

Take photos of your skin from different angles every few days or weekly. Visual proof can show changes that are not always noticeable on a daily basis. Ensure you take these photos in the same lighting conditions to track your progress more accurately.

3. Observe How Your Skin Reacts

Pay attention to how your skin feels after using certain remedies. Does your skin feel too dry, oily, or balanced? Reactions such as stinging, itching, or excessive dryness could be signs that a product is too harsh and needs adjusting. On the other hand, a softer, clearer complexion is a positive sign.

4. Be Patient with Natural Remedies

Natural acne treatments can take longer to show results, so give each remedy enough time to work, typically 4 to 6 weeks. If your skin isn't improving after this period, consider adjusting the ingredients or frequency of use. For example, if you're using tea tree oil, try reducing the concentration if your skin becomes irritated or increasing it if you see no results.

5. Adjust Based on Your Skin Type

Your skin type may influence how your skin reacts to natural treatments. For oily skin, you might want to focus on remedies that balance oil production, such as apple cider vinegar or witch hazel. For dry skin, ingredients like honey or aloe vera can provide moisture while treating acne. As you track your progress, notice if your skin becomes too dry or oily and adjust your regimen accordingly.

6. Review Your Diet and Lifestyle

Since diet and lifestyle play a big role in acne, take note of changes in your habits. For example, track what you eat, how much sleep you're getting, or how stressed you feel. These factors can affect your skin, so adjusting your diet by eating more fruits, vegetables, and water-rich foods may help with long-term improvement.

7. Consistency is Key

Track how consistently you are using your natural regimen. Inconsistent use can make it difficult to know if something is working. Sticking to a daily routine will provide a clearer picture of your progress.

8. Consult a Professional if Needed

If you've tracked your progress and see no improvement after a few months, it might be time to consult a dermatologist. They can provide guidance and suggest modifications to your natural regimen or alternative treatments.

By carefully observing and adjusting based on your skin's needs, you can ensure that your acne treatment is as effective as possible. Remember, the goal is to treat your skin gently and patiently, allowing natural remedies to work with your skin's healing process.

7.2 Tips for sustaining clear skin after acne treatment.

To sustain clear skin after acne treatment, especially when aiming for a natural approach, it's important to focus on habits that promote long-term skin health. **Here are some tips to help keep your skin clear and glowing:**

1. Follow a Consistent Skincare Routine

Maintain a simple yet effective skincare routine that includes gentle cleansing, toning, and moisturizing. Use products that are non-comedogenic (won't clog your pores), and avoid harsh chemicals. Look for natural ingredients like aloe vera and tea tree oil, which are known for their soothing and acne-fighting properties.

2. Stay Hydrated

Drinking plenty of water helps flush out toxins and keeps your skin hydrated. Proper hydration is essential for maintaining elasticity and preventing the buildup of impurities that can lead to breakouts.

3. Eat a Balanced Diet

What you eat affects your skin. Focus on eating fresh fruits, vegetables, and whole grains. Avoid processed foods, sugary snacks, and dairy, which are known to trigger acne in some people.

Incorporating foods rich in vitamins A, C, and E, along with omega-3 fatty acids, can help nourish the skin from the inside out.

4. Exfoliate Regularly but Gently

Regular exfoliation helps remove dead skin cells that can clog pores and cause breakouts. However, it's important to be gentle and not over-exfoliate. Using natural exfoliants like sugar scrubs or oatmeal once or twice a week can be enough to keep your skin smooth without irritation.

5. Manage Stress

Stress is a major trigger for acne, so finding ways to manage it is important. Engage in relaxation techniques such as deep breathing, yoga, or meditation. Getting sufficient sleep is crucial because it allows your skin to repair and rejuvenate.

6. Use Sunscreen Daily

Sun exposure can worsen acne scars and cause new breakouts. Always use a natural, oil-free sunscreen with SPF to protect your skin from harmful UV rays. This also prevents premature aging and helps maintain an even skin tone.

7. Avoid Touching Your Face

Your hands carry dirt and bacteria, which can transfer to your skin when you touch your face. Make it a habit to avoid picking at pimples or touching your skin unnecessarily to reduce the risk of breakouts and irritation.

8. Stay Active

Regular physical activity boosts blood circulation, helping to nourish skin cells and remove waste. However, always cleanse your skin after sweating to prevent clogged pores.

9. Choose Natural Remedies for Spot Treatment

If you notice a breakout starting, opt for natural spot treatments like diluted tea tree oil or a honey mask. These have antibacterial properties that can help reduce inflammation and prevent further breakouts.

10. Sleep Well

Your skin repairs itself while you sleep. Ensure you sleep very well for 7 to 8 hours every night.

Good sleep improves overall health and promotes a clear, glowing complexion.

By sticking to these tips, you can maintain clear skin naturally after acne treatment, allowing your skin to heal and thrive without relying on harsh chemicals.

Chapter 8

Natural Acne Treatments for Teens

8.1 Why teenage acne is different (hormones and puberty).

Teenage acne is a common issue that many young people face, and it differs from acne in adults primarily due to hormonal changes that occur during puberty. Understanding these differences can help in managing and treating acne effectively.

Hormonal Changes During Puberty

During puberty, the body undergoes significant hormonal shifts. The two main hormones involved in acne are:

1. Androgens: These are male hormones that both boys and girls produce. During puberty, the production of androgens increases, leading to several changes, such as:

- **Increased Oil Production:** Androgens stimulate the sebaceous glands in the skin to produce more oil (sebum). While some oil is necessary for healthy skin, too much can clog pores and lead to acne.

2. Estrogen: In girls, estrogen levels also rise during puberty. Although estrogen can help balance some of the effects of androgens, the initial spike in androgens often leads to an increase in acne.

Skin Changes

Alongside hormonal changes, the skin itself undergoes transformations during adolescence. Such as:

- **Thicker Skin:** The skin may become thicker during puberty, which can also contribute to clogged pores.
- **Increased Cell Turnover:** Young skin tends to regenerate faster, which can lead to more dead

skin cells accumulating in pores, further promoting acne.

Psychological Factors

Teenage years are not just about physical changes; they also bring emotional and psychological shifts. The stress of adolescence can exacerbate acne, as stress hormones can increase oil production and trigger breakouts.

Teenage acne is primarily driven by hormonal changes during puberty. Understanding these underlying factors can help teens and their caregivers choose appropriate treatments and manage expectations. While acne can be frustrating, it's a normal part of growing up and often improves with time and proper care.

8.2 Simple, budget-friendly natural skincare for teens.

Taking care of your skin doesn't have to be expensive or complicated. Here are some easy, natural skincare recipes that are perfect for teens.

These recipes use common ingredients that are gentle on the skin and easy to find.

1. Gentle Cleanser

Ingredients:

- 1 tablespoon honey
- 1 tablespoon plain yogurt
- 1 teaspoon lemon juice (optional)

Instructions:

1. In a small bowl, mix the honey and yogurt until smooth.
2. If desired, add lemon juice for its brightening properties.
3. Apply the mixture to your face, avoiding the eye area.
4. Let it sit for 5-10 minutes, then rinse with warm water.

2. Soothing Face Mask

Ingredients:

- 1 ripe banana
- 1 tablespoon oatmeal
- 1 tablespoon honey

Instructions:

1. Mash the banana in a bowl until smooth.
2. Add the oatmeal and honey, mixing until well combined.
3. Apply the mask to your face, allowing it to sit for 10-15 minutes.
4. Rinse off with warm water.

3. Moisturizing Lotion

Ingredients:

- 2 tablespoons coconut oil
- 1 tablespoon aloe vera gel
- A few drops of essential oil (like lavender or tea tree)

Instructions:

1. In a small bowl, combine coconut oil and aloe vera gel.
2. Add essential oil if desired for fragrance and skin benefits.
3. Mix well and store in a small jar.
4. Apply a small amount to your face after cleansing.

4. Exfoliating Scrub

Ingredients:

- 1 tablespoon sugar (brown or white)
- 1 tablespoon olive oil or coconut oil
- **Optional:** a few drops of lemon juice

Instructions:

1. In a bowl, mix the sugar and oil until it forms a paste.
2. If using, add lemon juice for extra brightness.

3. Gently massage the scrub onto your face in circular motions for about 1-2 minutes.
4. Rinse off with warm water. Use this scrub once a week.

5. Toner

Ingredients:

- 1 cup green tea (cooled)
- 1 tablespoon apple cider vinegar (optional)

Instructions:

1. Brew a cup of green tea and let it cool completely.
2. If desired, add apple cider vinegar for extra astringent properties.
3. Pour the mixture into a clean spray bottle.
4. Spray onto your face after cleansing, or apply with a cotton pad.

Tips for Healthy Skin

- **Remain Hydrated:** Make sure to consume plenty of water throughout the day.
- **Eat Well:** Incorporate fruits and vegetables into your diet for healthy skin.
- **Avoid Touching Your Face:** This can help reduce breakouts.
- **Wear Sunscreen:** Protect your skin from UV rays, even on cloudy days.

By using these simple, natural recipes, you can maintain healthy skin without breaking the bank. Enjoy your skincare routine!

8.3 Teen diet tips for balancing hormones and reducing breakouts.

Balancing hormones and reducing breakouts in teens often starts with a healthy diet. The right foods can help manage the natural hormonal changes that lead to acne. **Here are some teen diet tips for naturally balancing hormones and clearing up acne:**

1. Eat More Fruits and Vegetables

Fruits and vegetables are packed with vitamins, minerals, and antioxidants that support skin health. Vitamin C, found in oranges, berries, and leafy greens, is especially good for helping repair skin and reduce inflammation that can lead to breakouts. Try to eat a variety of colors, such as dark leafy greens like spinach, bright red tomatoes, and carrots rich in beta-carotene, which help maintain clear skin.

2. Choose Whole Grains Over Refined Carbs

Refined carbohydrates like white bread, pasta, and sugary snacks can spike blood sugar levels, which may cause a hormonal imbalance. This can trigger an increase in oil production, leading to clogged pores and acne. Switching to whole grains such as brown rice, oats, and whole wheat bread helps keep blood sugar levels steady, which supports hormonal balance.

3. Incorporate Healthy Fats

Healthy fats, like those found in avocados, olive oil, nuts, and seeds, are essential for hormone regulation. Omega-3 fatty acids, found in foods like salmon, chia seeds, and flaxseeds, are particularly helpful. These fats reduce inflammation in the skin, helping to calm redness and swelling from acne. Including a small amount of these fats in daily meals can make a big difference.

4. Limit Dairy Intake

Some studies suggest that dairy, particularly milk, can contribute to acne. This is because dairy products may contain hormones that can disrupt the body's natural hormonal balance. If dairy seems to worsen acne, try cutting back or choosing alternatives like almond, coconut, or oat milk.

5. Cut Back on Sugary Foods

Sugar causes blood sugar spikes, which in turn can increase the production of insulin. High insulin levels can lead to a surge in hormones that cause your skin to produce more oil. This excess oil can clog pores and lead to breakouts. Reducing sugary drinks like soda, and limiting candies and desserts can help keep skin clearer.

6. Stay Hydrated

Drinking enough water is key for healthy skin. Water helps flush toxins out of the body and keeps skin hydrated from the inside out. Proper hydration also helps balance oil production and can reduce the appearance of acne. Aim for at least 6-8 glasses of water a day to help keep skin looking its best.

7. Eat Foods Rich in Zinc

Zinc is an important mineral for skin health and hormone regulation. It helps reduce inflammation and prevents clogged pores. Foods high in zinc include pumpkin seeds, chickpeas, lentils, and nuts. Including zinc-rich foods in the diet may help reduce breakouts over time.

8. Balance Protein Intake

Teens need adequate protein for overall health, but it's important to choose the right types of protein. Lean proteins like chicken, turkey, fish, and plant-based sources like beans and lentils are better options than red meat, which can sometimes increase inflammation and trigger acne.

9. Avoid Processed Foods

Processed foods, such as chips, fast food, and ready-made meals, often contain unhealthy fats and preservatives that can upset hormone levels and contribute to acne. These foods are usually low in nutrients. Instead, focus on eating fresh, whole foods that nourish the body and skin.

10. Probiotics and Gut Health

A healthy gut can lead to healthier skin. Probiotics, found in foods like yogurt, kefir, and fermented vegetables like kimchi and sauerkraut, support gut health by balancing good bacteria in the digestive system. A balanced gut can help regulate hormones and reduce inflammation, which in turn can minimize breakouts.

Balancing hormones and reducing acne naturally is possible with the right dietary choices. Teens can support their skin health by eating a balanced diet rich in fruits, vegetables, whole grains, healthy fats, and lean proteins, while avoiding processed foods and too much sugar. Staying hydrated and including zinc and probiotics can further help maintain clear skin. These small changes can make a big difference in both how the skin looks and how balanced hormones feel.

www.ingramcontent.com/pod-product-compliance
Lightning Source LLC
Chambersburg PA
CBHW050309230526
45471CB00005B/2097